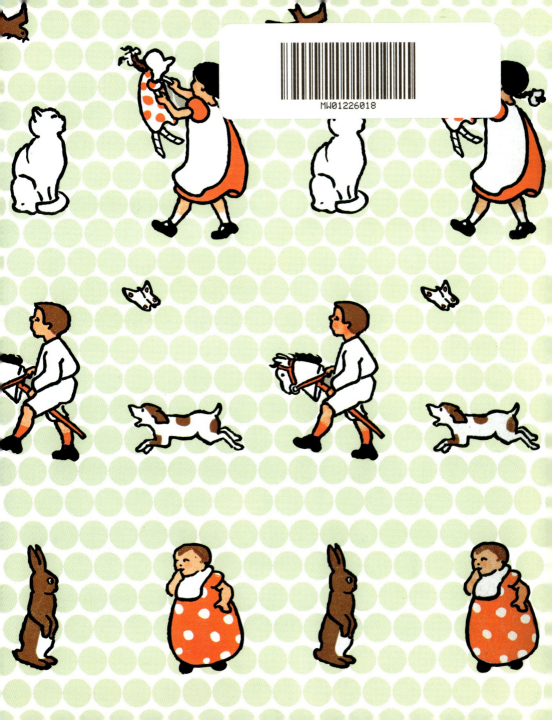

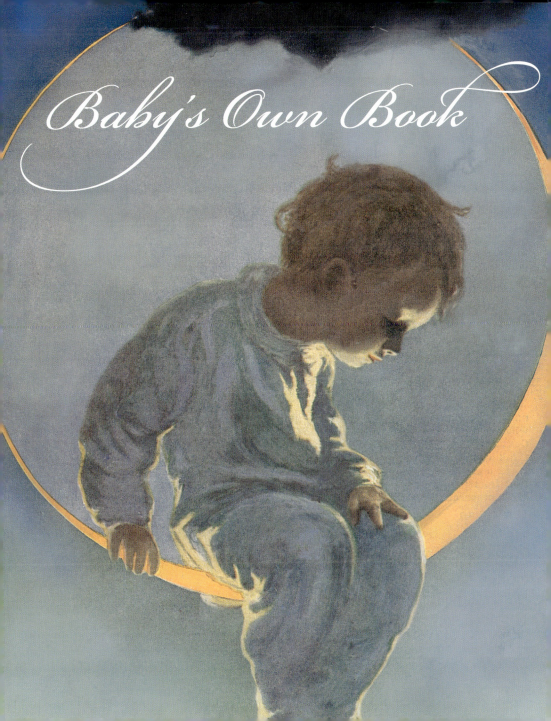

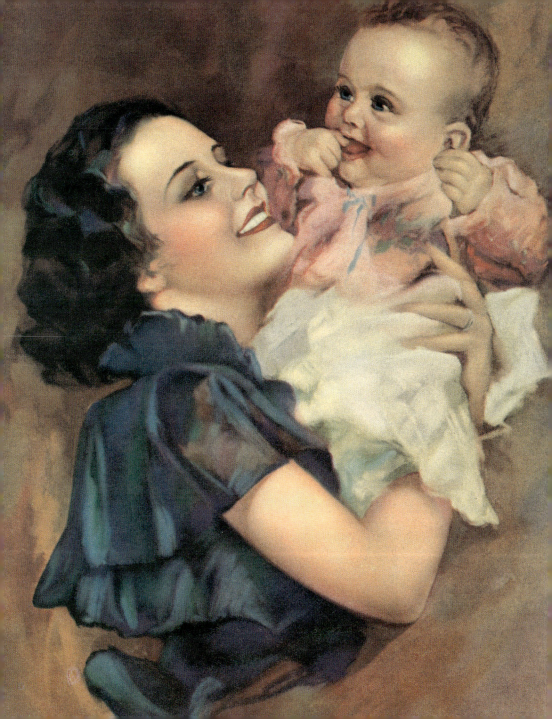

Baby's Own Book

Baby's First Year

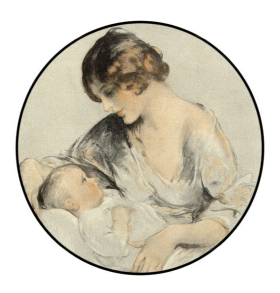

Compiled by Blue Lantern Studio

Laughing Elephant

MMIV

COPYRIGHT © 2004, BLUE LANTERN STUDIO

ISBN 1-883211-21-2

PRINTED IN CHINA THROUGH COLORCRAFT LTD., HONG KONG

LAUGHING ELEPHANT BOOKS

3645 INTERLAKE AVENUE NORTH   SEATTLE, WASHINGTON   98103

WWW.LAUGHINGELEPHANT.COM

The Baby Book Of:

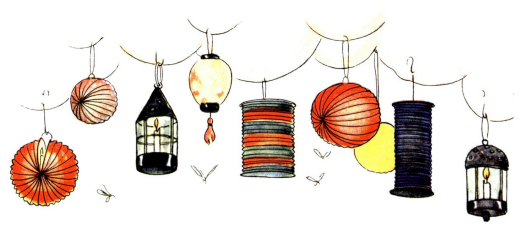

Name:

Birth date: Time:

Place:

City: State:

Parents:

Attendants:

Measurements:

Weight: Height:

Visitors...

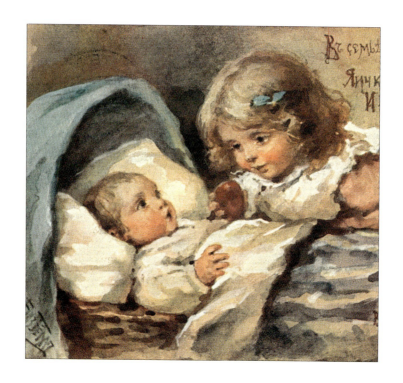

And What They Said

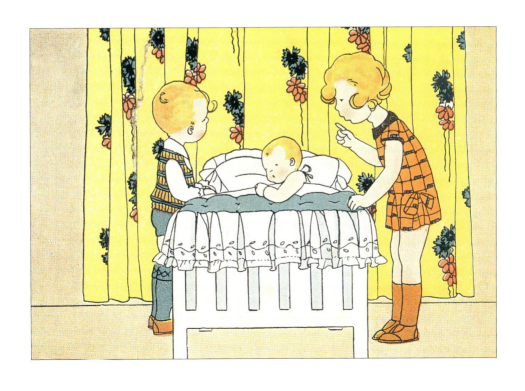

Measurements & Immunizations

Date: **Height:** **Weight:** **Immunizations:**

Gifts

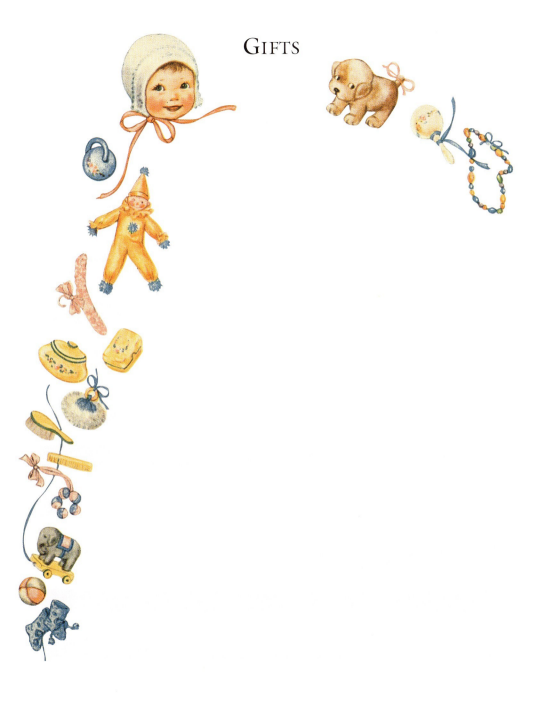

Baby Smiles

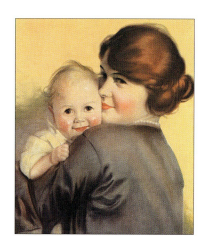

Date:

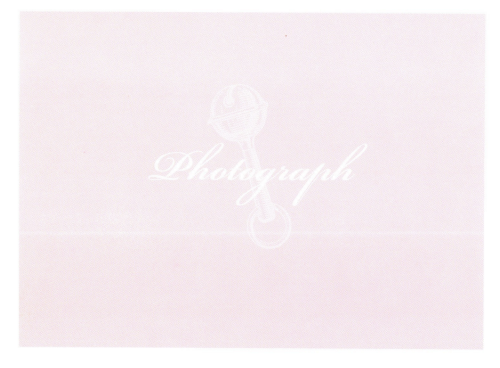

Baby's Bath

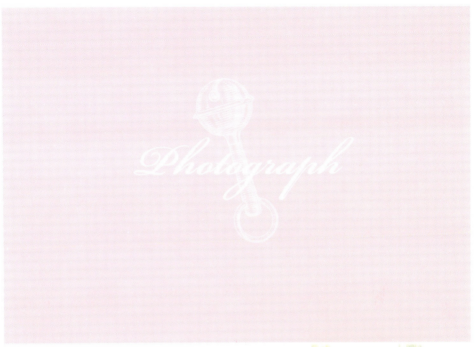

Date:

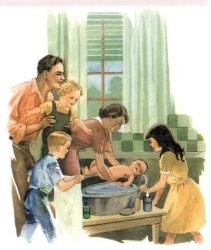

Baby's Friends

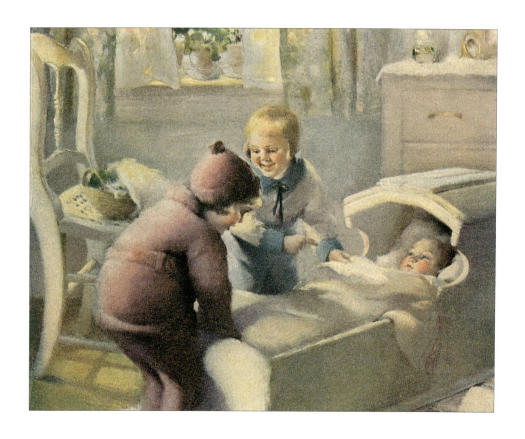

Baby's Friends

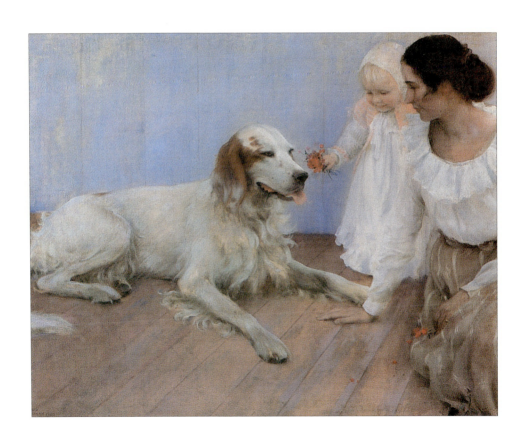

Baby Sits Up

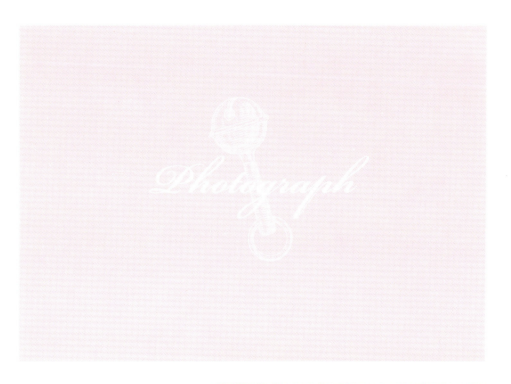

Date:

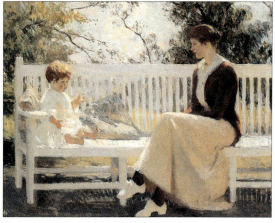

MILESTONES

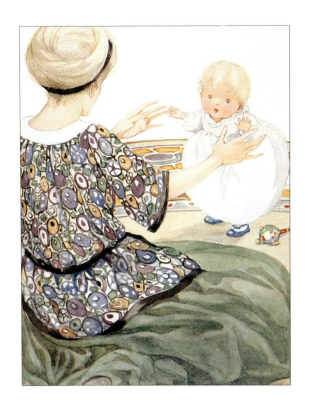

BABY CRAWLS • DATE:

BABY STANDS • DATE:

BABY WALKS • DATE:

Favorite Foods

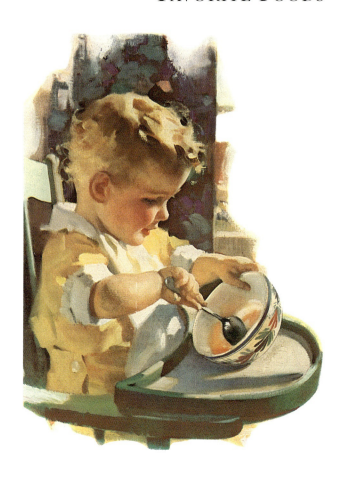

First Hair Cut

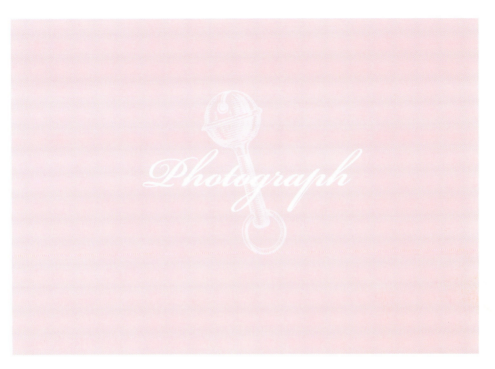

Date:

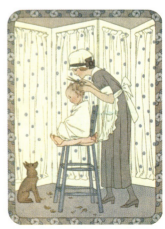

Lock of hair

Baby Speaks

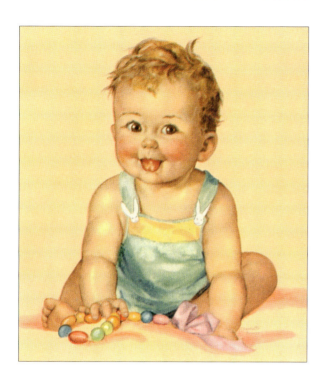

First Words:
1.
2.
3.
4.
5.
6.
7.
8.
9.
10.

Memorable sayings:

First Outing

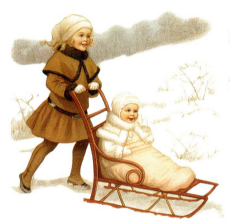

DATE:

WHERE:

Baby's Games & Toys

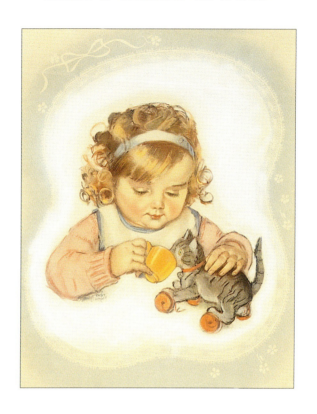

Favorite Outfit

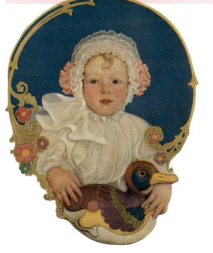

Date:

Holiday Memories

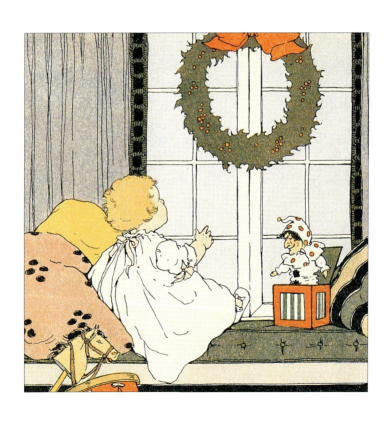

Baby's First Birthday

Date:

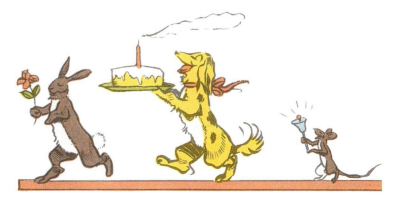

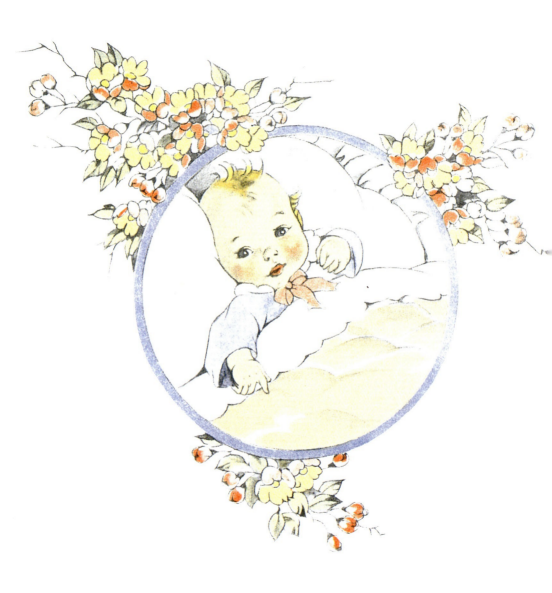

COVER	MAUD TOUSEY FANGEL. ILLUSTRATION, N.D.
ENDPAPERS	GERTRUDE CASPARI. FROM *KINDERLAND DU ZUBERLAND*, 1908.
HALF TITLE	VICTOR C. ANDERSON. MAGAZINE COVER, N.D.
FRONTISPIECE	UNKNOWN. CALENDAR ILLUSTRATION, N.D.
TITLE PAGE	GUY HOFF. MAGAZINE ILLUSTRATION, N.D.
PAGE 2	UNKNOWN. POSTCARD, N.D.
PAGE 3	CAMO. FROM *LA JOURNÉE DE BABY*, 1927.
PAGE 4	JANET LAURA SCOTT. FROM *BABYHOOD STEP BY STEP*, 1938.
PAGE 5	QUEEN HOLDEN. FROM *BABY'S RECORD*, 1929.
PAGE 6	UNKNOWN. ADVERTISEMENT, 1924.
PAGE 7	MILDRED LYON HETHERINGTON. FROM *GIRLS AND BOYS AND HOME*, 1955.
PAGE 8	NANA FRENCH BICKFORD. MAGAZINE COVER, 1911.
PAGE 9	CHARLES COURTNEY CURRAN. "ON THE PORCH," 1902.
PAGE 10	FRANK W. BENSON. "ELEANOR AND BENNY," 1916.
PAGE 11	ANNE ANDERSON. FROM *BABY'S RECORD*, 1920.
PAGE 12	UNKNOWN. ADVERTISEMENT, 1935.
PAGE 13	ANNE ANDERSON. FROM *BABY'S RECORD*, 1920.
PAGE 14	UNKNOWN. CALENDAR ILLUSTRATION, N.D.
PAGE 15	IDA A. WAUGH. FROM *WHEN MOTHER WAS A LITTLE GIRL*, N.D.
PAGE 16	MAUD TOUSEY FANGEL. FROM *BABIES*, 1941.
PAGE 17	SARAH STILWELL WEBER. MAGAZINE COVER, 1919.
PAGE 18	BLANCHE FISHER WRIGHT. FROM *BABY'S JOURNAL*, 1916.
PAGE 19	TONY SARG. FROM *BABY'S BOOK*, 1943.
PAGE 20	JANET LAURA SCOTT. FROM *BABYHOOD STEP BY STEP*, 1938.
BACK COVER	L. GODDARD. CALENDAR ILLUSTRATION, 1929.

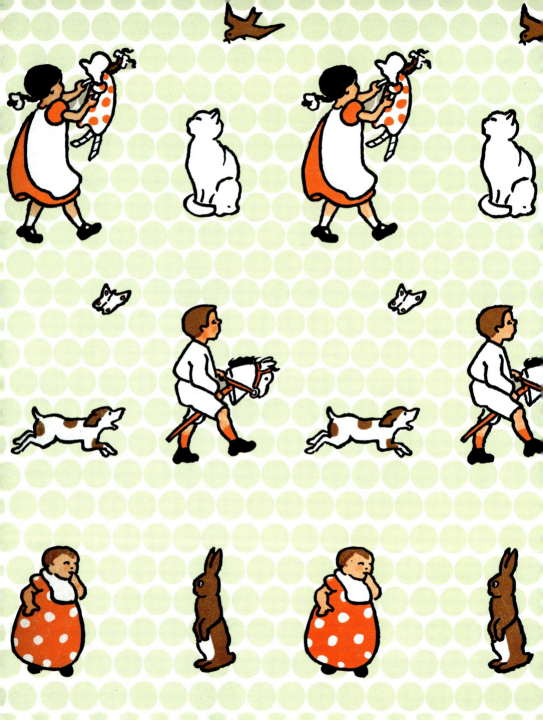